"Surviving Prostate: A Comprehensive Guide to Understanding, Preventing, and Thriving Beyond Cancer"

DISCLAIMER

The information contained in this resource is general in nature and for informative purposes only.

The Author assumes no responsibility whatsoever, under any circumstances, for any actions taken as a result of the information contained herein.

You are required to seek professional help if needed.

Preface

The shelves of bookstores are filled with many fine books on Prostate Cancer. Why another one? I believe there is always a need for simple truths – no matter how often they are told

The issue of Prostate Cancer has become a worrisome one to a lot of people suffering from this.

If by reading this book, a person can say" Wow, now I get it. I see something that could really help me*, then my purpose as an author has been fulfilled.

One of the greatest motivations in my own life is to see someone who has been dealing with a particular issue experience remarkable life change.

If I can help someone understand and apply the tips that he or she otherwise would have missed, then creating this book will have one of the most rewarding experience of my life.

LEO CHAMBERS

Introduction:

In the landscape of men's health, prostate cancer stands as a significant and often complex challenge. This book is a guide through the multifaceted terrain of prostate cancer, aiming to empower individuals with knowledge, support, and a comprehensive understanding of this prevalent condition.

As the second most common cancer affecting men worldwide, prostate cancer necessitates a closer look. This guide begins with an exploration of the basics, providing clarity on what prostate cancer is, its prevalence, and the impact it has on individuals and their families. By establishing this foundational knowledge, we lay the groundwork for informed decision-making and proactive health management.

Our journey continues by delving into the various factors that contribute to the development of prostate cancer. From genetic predispositions to the influence of lifestyle and environmental factors, we unravel the intricate tapestry that makes some individuals more susceptible to this condition than others.

Early detection becomes a focal point, with an examination of screening methods such as the PSA test and digital rectal exams. Through this exploration, readers will gain insights into the importance of timely diagnosis and the potential benefits and risks associated with screening.

Moving forward, we navigate the complexities of different types and stages of prostate cancer. Understanding these nuances is crucial for individuals facing treatment decisions, whether it be active surveillance, surgery, radiation therapy, or emerging approaches like immunotherapy.

This book is not just a clinical guide; it's a companion for the emotional and psychological aspects of the prostate cancer journey. We address the challenges, provide coping strategies, and offer support for patients and their families, recognizing the holistic nature of the impact of prostate cancer on individuals' lives.

As we progress, we shine a light on survivorship, emphasizing the importance of life after treatment and the ongoing pursuit of a high quality of life. This journey is complemented by a discussion on prevention strategies, encouraging lifestyle modifications and proactive health measures.

In conclusion, this guide is designed to be a beacon of knowledge, support, and encouragement for those navigating the complexities of prostate cancer. By providing comprehensive insights and practical advice, we aim to empower individuals to face the challenges of prostate cancer with resilience and informed decision-making.

Table of Contents

Chapter 10 - Advances in Prostate Cancer Research

Conclusion

Chapter 1

Understanding Prostate Cancer

Prostate Cancer: Definition, Description, and Insights

Prostate cancer is a significant health concern affecting men worldwide, characterized by the abnormal growth of cells in the prostate gland, a vital component of the male reproductive system. This comprehensive exploration delves into the definition, epidemiology, etiology, pathophysiology, clinical manifestations, diagnosis, staging, treatment modalities, prognosis, and preventive strategies associated with prostate cancer.

Prostate cancer manifests as the uncontrolled proliferation of malignant cells within the prostate gland, a walnut-sized organ located beneath the bladder and surrounding the urethra. As the second most common cancer in men globally, prostate cancer presents diverse clinical manifestations, ranging from indolent, low-grade tumors to aggressive, high-risk disease variants.

Epidemiology:

Prostate cancer predominately affects older men, with the majority of cases diagnosed after the age of 50. The incidence varies geographically, with higher rates observed in North America, Europe, and Australia, while lower rates are reported in Asia and Africa. Risk factors include age, family history, ethnicity, genetic predisposition, and lifestyle factors such as diet, physical activity, and exposure to environmental carcinogens.

Etiology and Pathophysiology:

The etiology of prostate cancer is multifactorial, involving genetic, hormonal, environmental, and lifestyle influences. Genetic mutations, alterations in androgen receptor signaling pathways, inflammation, and oxidative stress contribute to the initiation and progression of prostate cancer. Dysregulation of cell cycle control mechanisms, apoptosis, DNA repair processes, and angiogenesis play pivotal roles in tumor development and metastasis.

Clinical Manifestations:

Prostate cancer often presents asymptomatically in its early stages, making early detection challenging. As the disease progresses, symptoms may include urinary dysfunction (e.g., frequency, urgency, nocturia, hesitancy, weak stream), hematuria, erectile dysfunction, pelvic pain, bone pain, and systemic manifestations such as weight loss and fatigue. However, these symptoms are nonspecific and may mimic benign prostatic hyperplasia (BPH) or other urological conditions.

Diagnosis:

The diagnosis of prostate cancer relies on a multidisciplinary approach, incorporating clinical evaluation, digital rectal examination (DRE), serum prostate-specific antigen (PSA) testing, imaging studies (e.g., transrectal ultrasound, magnetic resonance imaging), and prostate biopsy. PSA levels, prostate volume, age, and patient risk factors inform decision-making regarding the need for further diagnostic evaluation and biopsy.

Staging and Risk Stratification:

Prostate cancer staging utilizes the tumor, node, metastasis (TNM) classification system, assessing tumor size, extent of local invasion, lymph node involvement, and distant metastases. Risk stratification integrates clinical, pathological, and molecular features to categorize patients into low, intermediate, high, and very high-risk groups, guiding treatment selection and prognosis estimation.

Treatment Modalities:

Prostate cancer management encompasses a spectrum of treatment modalities tailored to individual patient characteristics, disease stage, aggressiveness, and patient preferences. Options include active surveillance, radical prostatectomy, radiation therapy (external beam, brachytherapy), androgen deprivation therapy (ADT), chemotherapy, immunotherapy, targeted therapies, and palliative care interventions. Treatment decisions prioritize oncologic outcomes, quality of life considerations, and potential treatment-related side effects.

Prognosis:

Prostate cancer prognosis varies widely based on disease stage, grade, histological subtype, molecular biomarkers, and treatment response. The majority of prostate cancers are localized at diagnosis, with favorable long-term outcomes following curative-intent therapy. However, advanced or metastatic disease poses significant challenges, necessitating multimodal treatment approaches and palliative care interventions to optimize quality of life and survival outcomes.

Preventive Strategies:

Prostate cancer prevention strategies encompass lifestyle modifications, dietary interventions, regular exercise, smoking cessation, moderation of alcohol consumption, weight management, screening guidelines, genetic counseling, and chemoprevention agents (e.g., 5-alpha-reductase inhibitors). Shared decision-making between patients and healthcare providers facilitates informed choices regarding screening, early detection, and risk reduction strategies.

In summary, prostate cancer represents a complex and multifaceted disease entity with diverse clinical presentations, diagnostic challenges, treatment considerations, and prognostic implications. This comprehensive overview underscores the importance of interdisciplinary collaboration, patient-centered care, ongoing research endeavors, and public health initiatives in combating prostate cancer and improving patient outcomes. Through continued efforts in prevention, early detection, treatment innovation, and survivorship support, we endeavor to mitigate the burden of prostate cancer and enhance the quality of life for individuals affected by this prevalent malignancy.

Regular screenings are recommended for men over the age of 50, or earlier for those with a family history of the disease. Screening tests, such as the prostate-specific antigen (PSA) test and digital rectal exam, are used to detect the presence of prostate cancer in its early stages when treatment is most effective.

Early detection can lead to more successful treatment outcomes and improved survival rates for individuals diagnosed with prostate cancer. It is important for men to discuss their risk factors and screening options with their healthcare provider to determine the best course of action for their individual effectiveness.

In addition to genetic factors, hormonal influences, and environmental/lifestyle factors, screening and early detection play a crucial role in understanding and managing prostate cancer.

Survivorship and quality of life post-treatment are equally important considerations. Completing treatment marks the beginning of survivorship, and regular follow-up care, including medical check-ups and screenings, is crucial.

Additionally, making lifestyle adjustments, such as maintaining a healthy diet and engaging in regular exercise, can greatly contribute to enhanced well-being post-treatment.

In conclusion, understanding prostate cancer requires a comprehensive exploration of its genetic, hormonal, and environmental influences. Effective screening methods, a range of treatment options, considerations for emotional well-being, survivorship, ongoing research, and prevention strategies all equip individuals and their support networks with the tools needed to navigate the prostate cancer journey with resilience and informed decision-making.

Prostate cancer can display varying degrees of aggressiveness. The Gleason score, a grading system, helps categorize the aggressiveness of the cancer based on the appearance of cells under a microscope.

Additionally, staging through the TNM system is employed to evaluate the extent of cancer spread, guiding treatment decisions. Advances in prostate cancer research offer promising treatment innovations.

Ongoing research explores novel therapies, targeted treatments, and advancements in precision medicine. Investigating the genetic basis of prostate cancer and exploring immunotherapeutic approaches hold promise for future breakthroughs.

Prevention strategies are an integral part of prostate health. Lifestyle modifications, such as following a balanced diet rich in fruits and vegetables and low in saturated fats, along with regular exercise, can contribute to overall prostate health.

Individuals with a family history of prostate cancer may also consider genetic counseling and testing to assess their risk and make informed decisions. Early detection plays a critical role in effectively managing prostate cancer.

Screening methods, such as the Prostate-Specific Antigen (PSA) blood test and digital rectal exams, are utilized to identify potential issues. The PSA test measures the levels of a protein produced by the prostate, which can indicate the presence of cancer.

However, it is important to note that elevated PSA levels are not a definitive diagnostic tool on their own. When it comes to treating prostate cancer, the approach taken depends on several factors, including the stage of cancer, the age of the patient, and their overall health.

Treatment options encompass a variety of approaches, such as active surveillance, surgery (radical prostatectomy), radiation therapy, hormone therapy, and advanced treatments like chemotherapy and immunotherapy for more aggressive cases.

Support groups and resources play a vital role in providing emotional support and shared experiences for patients and their families. Recognizing the vital role of caregivers and addressing their unique challenges is also crucial for comprehensive patient care.

Living with prostate cancer can be emotionally challenging. Coping with the diagnosis requires support systems, counseling, and education about the disease to help individuals adapt to their new reality.

Managing treatment side effects is also an important aspect of maintaining a good quality of life, as various treatments may have side effects such as urinary incontinence or sexual dysfunction.

Understanding the complexities of genetic, hormonal, and environmental influences on prostate cancer is crucial. Coupled with effective screening methods and a range of treatment options, this knowledge forms the foundation for navigating the landscape of prostate cancer.

It empowers individuals and healthcare professionals to make informed decisions regarding prevention, early detection, and personalized treatment plans.

Chapter 2

Causes of Prostate Cancer

There are also racial and ethnic disparities when it comes to prostate cancer risk factors. Studies have shown that African American men have a higher incidence and mortality rate from prostate cancer compared to men of other racial and ethnic backgrounds.

The reasons for this disparity are complex and may involve a combination of genetic, environmental, and socioeconomic factors. Additionally, research has indicated that men of Asian descent may have a lower risk of developing prostate cancer compared to men of other ethnicities. Understanding and addressing these disparities is crucial in order to improve outcomes for all individuals affected by prostate cancer.

Lifestyle and environmental factors also contribute to the varying rates of prostate cancer among different ethnic background.

Dietary habits, for instance, play a role in prostate cancer risk. African American diets, which are often high in red meat and low in fruits and vegetables, have been associated with an increased likelihood of developing prostate cancer.

In contrast, Asian diets, rich in plant-based foods and green tea, have been linked to a lower risk of the disease. Additionally, exposure to environmental toxins and pollutants, such as those found in certain occupations or residential areas, may also contribute to the disparities in prostate cancer rates.

These lifestyle and environmental factors serve as additional layers to the complex puzzle of prostate cancer disparities, emphasizing the need for comprehensive prevention strategies.

Hormonal factors also contribute to the disparities in prostate cancer rates among different ethnic groups. Testosterone, the primary male sex hormone, has been linked to the development and progression of prostate cancer. African American men tend to have higher levels of testosterone compared to other racial groups, which may explain their increased susceptibility to the disease.

On the other hand, Asian populations have been found to have lower testosterone levels, potentially contributing to their decreased risk of developing prostate cancer. These hormonal variations highlight the intricate interplay between genetics and hormones in prostate cancer occurrence.

Prostate Intraepithelial Neoplasia (PIN) refers to the presence of abnormal cells within the prostate gland, which may indicate an increased risk for developing prostate cancer.

To fully comprehend the causes of prostate cancer, a comprehensive and holistic approach is required. This involves considering both intrinsic factors, such as genetics and hormones, and extrinsic factors, such as environmental exposures and lifestyle choices.

By understanding the intricate interplay between these various factors, we can lay a strong foundation for developing targeted prevention strategies, personalized treatment plans, and fostering ongoing research to unravel the complexities of this prevalent cancer.

Prostate Intraepithelial Neoplasia (PIN) is considered a precursor lesion for prostate cancer, specifically high-grade PIN, which is linked to an increased risk of developing invasive cancer. The significance of identifying PIN in prostate biopsies cannot be understated, as it prompts closer monitoring and proactive management to prevent the progression of the disease.

The task at hand requires a significantly greater amount of effort and dedication in order to achieve the desired outcome.

The complexity and scope of the project demand a higher level of commitment and perseverance in order to successfully navigate the challenges and obstacles that may arise.

It is imperative to approach the task with a mindset of determination and resilience, as the road ahead is filled with twists and turns that will test our abilities and resolve. Only through unwavering perseverance and a steadfast dedication to the task at hand can we hope to overcome the hurdles and achieve our ultimate goal.

It is crucial to maintain a positive attitude and a strong work ethic in order to push through the inevitable setbacks that may come our way. By staying focused and committed to the task, we can ensure that we are able to overcome any challenges and emerge victorious in the end.

Chapter 3

Screening And Early Detection

In addition to the PSA test and DRE, imaging tests such as MRI or ultrasound may be used to further evaluate the prostate and aid in the diagnosis and staging of prostate cancer.

These tests can provide detailed images of the prostate gland, helping healthcare providers assess the extent of the disease and plan appropriate treatment interventions.

A digital rectal exam involves a physical examination of the prostate through the rectum to check for abnormalities in size, shape, or texture. This exam is often performed in conjunction with the PSA test to enhance the accuracy of early detection and provide a more comprehensive assessment of prostate health.

Moreover, early detection through timely screenings can help prevent the progression of prostate cancer to advanced stages, where treatment options may be limited and outcomes less favorable.

By detecting the disease early, individuals have a greater chance of receiving curative treatment and maintaining a higher quality of life following diagnosis.

The PSA test is a commonly used screening method for prostate cancer that measures the level of prostate-specific antigen in the blood. Elevated PSA levels can indicate various prostate conditions, including cancer, but it is important to note that PSA levels can also be influenced by other factors.

Despite some controversy surrounding its effectiveness, the PSA test remains a valuable tool in the early detection of prostate cancer. Early detection plays a crucial role in improving treatment outcomes for individuals diagnosed with prostate cancer.

By identifying the disease at an early stage, healthcare providers can implement more effective treatment strategies and increase the chances of successful outcomes.

Additionally, early detection allows for the distinction between slow-growing and aggressive forms of prostate cancer, enabling healthcare providers to tailor treatment plans accordingly and provide personalized care to patients.

Navigating these challenges and controversies requires a balanced approach that takes into account individual risk factors, preferences, and discussions with healthcare professionals.

It is important for individuals to be informed about the potential benefits and risks of screening and to engage in shared decision-making with their healthcare providers. By considering all factors and staying up-to-date on emerging technologies and biomarkers, individuals can make informed choices about their prostate cancer screening.

The dilemma of over diagnosis in prostate cancer screening involves the challenge of distinguishing between cancers that will never cause harm and those that require intervention.

This dilemma is further complicated by concerns regarding overtreatment, as treating cancers that are not aggressive can lead to unnecessary side effects.

To address these issues, public awareness and education initiatives are important in promoting informed decision-making. These initiatives aim to raise awareness about prostate cancer, the significance of screening, and the importance of making informed choices about one's health.

Additionally, advancements in imaging technologies, such as prostate-specific PET scans, are being developed to improve the accuracy of detecting and staging prostate cancer. Ongoing research on biomarkers and genetic testing may also provide more precise indications of prostate cancer risk and aggressiveness.

In conclusion, the field of prostate cancer screening and early detection is constantly evolving, with new technologies, recommendations, and discussions shaping the approach to managing this disease. A patient-centered approach, shared decision-making, and staying informed about emerging advancements are crucial components of effectively managing prostate cancer from its early stages.

Chapter 4

Types And Stages of Prostate Cancer

The Gleason score plays a crucial role in determining the aggressiveness of prostate cancer. This score, obtained from biopsy samples, evaluates the appearance of cancer cells and ranges from 6 (indicating low-grade cancer) to 10 (indicating high-grade cancer).

Ative surveillance involves close monitoring of low-risk prostate cancer through regular check-ups, PSA tests, and occasional biopsies. Watchful waiting, a conservative approach, may be suitable for older patients or those with significant comorbidities. Low-risk prostate cancer is characterized by a low Gleason score, smaller tumor size, and lower PSA levels, making active surveillance a suitable approach for many patients.

Intermediate and high-risk prostate cancer, with higher Gleason scores, larger tumors, and elevated PSA levels, may require more aggressive treatments like surgery or radiation.

Precision medicine and clinical trials are exploring novel treatments and therapeutic combinations to advance prostate cancer care and target specific genetic mutations.

Multiparametric MRI and PET scans, such as PSMA-PET scans, offer detailed images of the prostate, aiding in tumor visualization and assessing cancer aggressiveness.

Treatment options for localized, locally advanced, and metastatic prostate cancer include surgery, radiation therapy, hormone therapy, chemotherapy, and immunotherapy, tailored to the specific stage of the cancer.

The TNM staging system categorizes prostate cancer based on the extent of the primary tumor within the prostate (T), whether cancer has spread to nearby lymph nodes (N), and if cancer has metastasized to distant organs or tissues (M).

Stages range from I (localized cancer) to IV (advanced cancer with potential distant spread).

Prostate cancer is categorized into low-risk and high-risk groups based on factors like the Gleason score, PSA levels, and the extent of cancer, which helps in making informed decisions about treatment options.

Palliative care focuses on improving the quality of life for individuals with advanced prostate cancer, addressing symptoms and providing emotional support.

It can be integrated alongside active treatments to enhance overall well-being. Genomic testing helps identify specific mutations in prostate cancer cells, guiding treatment decisions and predicting response to therapies.

Targeted therapies that target specific molecular pathways in prostate cancer cells are emerging as more precise and effective treatment options. Follow-up care and addressing quality of life issues, such as sexual function, urinary and bowel habits, and emotional well-being, are essential aspects of survivorship care for individuals with prostate cancer.

The Gleason score combines the two most common patterns seen in prostate cancer tissue, providing a comprehensive evaluation of cancer aggressiveness. A higher Gleason score indicates a higher risk of cancer progression and can influence treatment decisions.

Chapter 5

Prevention Strategies

Support Groups: Promote the involvement in support groups for individuals diagnosed with prostate cancer or for those at high risk, providing a space for sharing experiences, gaining knowledge, and receiving emotional support.

 Risk-Benefit Analysis: Discuss the potential benefits and risks of hormone therapy for individuals at high risk of developing aggressive prostate cancer.

Prioritizing Quality Sleep: Highlight the importance of getting enough sleep and maintaining regular sleep patterns to support overall health and potentially reduce the risk of prostate cancer.

Water as a Primary Beverage: Promote water as the main beverage choice, limiting the intake of sugary drinks that have been linked to various health issues, including an increased risk of cancer.

 Educational Programs: Organize educational programs and workshops to raise awareness about prostate cancer prevention strategies, risk factors, and the importance of early detection.

Investment in Research: Emphasize the need for ongoing research to better understand the causes of prostate cancer, identify new prevention strategies, and improve treatment options.

By implementing these comprehensive prevention strategies and promoting awareness at individual, community, and societal levels, we can make significant progress in reducing the burden of prostate cancer and improving overall health outcomes.

Open Communication: Encourage individuals to establish a collaborative relationship with their healthcare providers, discussing any concerns, and actively participating in their healthcare decisions.

Clinical Trials: Encourage individuals to consider participating in clinical trials to contribute to the advancement of prostate cancer prevention and treatment.

Legislation Support: Advocate for policies that promote cancer prevention initiatives, such as increased access to screenings, education, and support services.

Individualized Treatment Plan: Encourage individuals to consult with their healthcare provider to determine if hormone therapy is a suitable option for managing their risk.

Regular Check-ups: Stress the importance of regular check-ups and screenings as part of a proactive approach to prostate cancer prevention.

Maintaining Adequate Fluid Intake: Stress the importance of staying properly hydrated to support overall health and potentially reduce the risk of prostate cancer.

Establishing a bedtime Routine: Encourage individuals to establish a consistent bedtime routine that promotes relaxation and better sleep quality.

Funding Allocation: Support efforts to allocate sufficient funding for research and programs aimed at prostate cancer prevention and early detection.

Addressing Disparities: Work collectively to address global disparities in access to preventive healthcare and cancer screenings, aiming to ensure equal opportunities for all individuals.

International Partnerships: Foster collaborations between countries to facilitate the sharing of knowledge, resources, and best practices in the prevention of prostate cancer.

Supportive Work Environments: Create work environments that support employees in maintaining a healthy work-life balance, reducing stressors, and fostering overall well-being.

Public Education Campaigns: Conduct campaigns to educate the public about preventive measures and lifestyle choices related to prostate cancer, ensuring that up-to-date information is disseminated.

 Accessible Health Resources: Provide easily accessible resources within communities for individuals to access regular health check-ups, screenings, and receive lifestyle counseling.

Nutrition and Health Policies: Support public policies that promote healthier food options and discourage the consumption of processed and unhealthy foods, aiming to improve overall nutrition and health.

 Water Consumption: Encourage individuals to regularly consume water as part of a well-rounded and healthy lifestyle, potentially contributing to overall well-being

Promoting Health at Work: Collaborate with employers to establish workplace wellness programs that promote healthy habits and encourage employees to prioritize regular health check-ups.

Education and Outreach Programs: Implement initiatives within communities to raise awareness about the risk factors associated with prostate cancer and the importance of preventive measures.

Investment in Research: Promote ongoing research efforts focused on preventing prostate cancer, exploring new insights, and developing innovative strategies.

Tobacco Control Policies: Advocate for and support policies aimed at controlling tobacco use and implementing effective smoking cessation programs.

Individualized Counseling: Offer personalized risk assessment and counseling services, taking into account individual factors such as age, family history, and genetic predispositions to prostate cancer.

Limiting Sugary Beverages: Advocate for the reduction of sugary drinks and encourage individuals to replace them with healthier alternatives such as water, herbal teas, or low-calorie beverages.

Tailored Prevention Plans: Develop tailored prevention plans based on individual risk profiles and health needs.

In conclusion, the prevention of prostate cancer requires a comprehensive and collaborative effort from individuals, healthcare providers, communities, and policymakers.

By incorporating these strategies into daily life, promoting awareness, and advocating for supportive environments, we can collectively work towards reducing the incidence and impact of prostate cancer on a global scale.

Chapter 6

Treatment Options

Targeted therapies, like Abiraterone and Enzalutamide, focus on specific molecules involved in cancer growth and may be used in advanced cases or when other treatments are ineffective.

Palliative care aims to address symptoms, provide emotional support, and enhance overall quality of life for individuals with advanced prostate cancer, while integrative and complementary therapies like nutritional counseling and mindfulness may complement traditional treatments.

Precision medicine and genomic testing analyze the genetic makeup of prostate cancer cells to guide treatment decisions, especially valuable in advanced or metastatic cases where targeted therapies may be more effective.

Follow-up care and survivorship plans involve regular monitoring, addressing quality of life considerations, and tailoring long-term plans for survivorship.

 Overall, understanding the diverse array of treatment options empowers individuals and healthcare teams to make informed decisions based on the specific characteristics of the prostate cancer, its stage, and the individual's overall health.

Collaboration among specialists, ongoing research, advances in precision medicine, and a holistic approach to well-being all contribute to optimizing care and outcomes for individuals facing prostate cancer at various stages of their journey.

Active surveillance is often recommended for low-risk prostate cancer cases, where the cancer is slow-growing and may not pose an immediate threat. This approach involves regular check-ups, PSA tests, and occasional biopsies to monitor any changes in cancer progression. The goal is to avoid the potential side effects of more aggressive treatments while still having the option for intervention if the cancer shows signs of progression.

Clinical trials investigate novel treatments and technologies, offering access to cutting-edge therapies and contributing to advancements in prostate cancer care. Personalized decision-making involves collaborative discussions among healthcare providers and considering individual risk profiles to tailor treatment decisions to each patient's unique needs.

.Hormoneherapy, also known as androgen deprivation therapy (ADT), aims to reduce testosterone levels to slow down cancer growth. It is used in various stages of prostate cancer, including before surgery or radiation and for advanced or metastatic cases, but can lead to side effects like hot flashes, fatigue, and potential long-term effects on bone health.

 Chemotherapy targets rapidly dividing cancer cells and is typically used in advanced or metastatic cases, while immunotherapy stimulates the immune system to recognize and attack cancer cells, often in advanced stages or as part of clinical trials.

Both treatments come with their own set of side effects, such as nausea, fatigue, and immune-related reactions.

Supportive care and well-being measures, including psychosocial support and physical wellness strategies, help address the emotional and physical impact of a prostate cancer diagnosis and enhance overall well-being during and after treatment.

 In advanced stages, shared decision-making, end-of-life care discussions, and advanced care planning are crucial in determining the most appropriate treatment strategy and respecting individual wishes.

 When it comes to treating prostate cancer, there is a wide range of options available to patients and their healthcare teams. These options include active surveillance, surgery, radiation therapy, hormone therapy, chemotherapy, immunotherapy, targeted therapies, palliative care, integrative and complementary therapies, precision medicine and genomic testing, follow-up care and survivorship plans, participation in clinical trials, personalized decision-making, and supportive care and well-being measures.

Radiation therapy, either through external beam radiation or brachytherapy, targets cancer cells with high-energy beams and radioactive seeds placed directly into the prostate. This treatment is often used for localized or locally advanced prostate cancer and may result in side effects such as fatigue, urinary changes, and bowel irritation.

Surgery, specifically radical prostatectomy, involves the complete removal of the prostate gland and surrounding tissues for localized prostate cancer cases.

However, this procedure may come with potential side effects such as erectile dysfunction and urinary incontinence post-surgery.

Chapter 7

Living With Prostate Cancer

Receiving a prostate cancer diagnosis can trigger a wide range of emotions that are important to acknowledge and address in order to maintain overall well-being.

Building a strong support system consisting of family, friends, and healthcare professionals can help individuals navigate the emotional challenges that come with a cancer diagnosis.

Life after cancer treatment involves adapting to changes and focusing on overall health and well-being. Regular follow-up care, check-ups, and screenings are essential to monitor for potential recurrence or long-term side effects.

Embracing a new normal and actively working towards a fulfilling and healthy life are important aspects of survivorship after prostate cancer treatment.

Many individuals may experience erectile dysfunction following surgery or radiation treatment for prostate cancer. It is important to communicate openly with healthcare providers and explore various treatment options to address this issue.

Additionally, managing urinary changes such as incontinence or alterations in urinary habits may involve pelvic floor exercises or other interventions. Fatigue is a common side effect of cancer treatment, and integrating strategies like regular exercise and seeking emotional support can help individuals manage their overall well-being during this time.

Anxiety and depression are common concerns for individuals dealing with a prostate cancer diagnosis. Routine screenings for these mental health issues are crucial, and seeking counseling, joining support groups, and practicing mindfulness techniques can be beneficial in managing these emotions.

Addressing sexual health concerns through open communication with healthcare providers and exploring available options can also help individuals cope with the psychological impact of their diagnosis and treatment.

In addition to individual support, it is important for patients and their families to have access to resources and support systems that can help them navigate the challenges of a prostate cancer diagnosis and treatment.

Providing support for both the patient and their loved ones can contribute to a more positive and empowered experience throughout the cancer journey.

Maintaining a balanced diet rich in fruits, vegetables, and whole grains, as well as engaging in regular physical activity, can support overall health and well-being for individuals dealing with prostate cancer.

Lifestyle modifications such as smoking cessation and moderation in alcohol consumption can also play a role in improving health outcomes and quality of life.

Being part of support groups allows individuals to connect with others facing similar challenges, creating a sense of community and shared experiences.

Accessing educational resources empowers individuals and families to make informed decisions. Recognizing the important role of caregivers and addressing their unique challenges is crucial for comprehensive patient care.

Coping strategies such as mindfulness and relaxation techniques can help alleviate stress, while education and advocacy can enhance a sense of control.

Building resilience involves adapting to challenges, seeking support, and maintaining a positive outlook. Open communication with healthcare providers fosters collaboration in care, addressing concerns and making informed decisions.

End-of-life planning and support, fertility discussions, financial considerations, continued health monitoring, and the impact on relationships are all important aspects of managing prostate cancer.

Active participation in supportive programs and community engagement can enhance overall quality of life.

Embracing Positivity and Hope:

Mindset Shift: Adopting a positive mindset and cultivating hope contribute to resilience during the prostate cancer journey.

Celebrating Milestones: Acknowledging and celebrating treatment milestones and personal achievements enhances the sense of accomplishment.

Living with prostate cancer is a dynamic journey that requires a multidimensional approach. Embracing ongoing health monitoring, open communication, and a proactive stance towards well-being fosters a positive and empowered life after diagnosis.

Individual experiences may vary, but the collective efforts of healthcare providers, support networks, and the individuals themselves contribute to a meaningful and fulfilling life with prostate cancer.

Chapter 8

Survivorship And Quality of Life

Holistic Approach: Taking a holistic approach to survivorship by addressing physical, emotional, and spiritual needs through a combination of conventional and complementary treatments.

Empowerment Through Advocacy: Advocating for oneself in the healthcare system to ensure personalized and comprehensive care.

Continued Education: Staying informed about advancements in cancer research, treatment options, and survivorship resources to make informed decisions about one's health.

Finding Meaning: Reflecting on the experience of cancer and finding ways to derive meaning, purpose, and growth from the challenges faced during treatment and beyond.

Building a Support System: Engaging with family, friends, and support groups to navigate the challenges of survivorship and receive emotional support.

Incorporating Integrative and Complementary Therapies: Exploring alternative therapies such as acupuncture, massage, and mindfulness practices to enhance overall well-being and manage symptoms.

Peer Networks: Connecting with other cancer survivors to share experiences, advice, and encouragement in a safe and understanding environment.

Acknowledging Achievements: Recognizing and celebrating milestones in the survivorship journey, whether big or small.

Exploring a variety of holistic approaches, such as acupuncture and yoga, to improve overall well-being is a key aspect of survivorship.

 Additionally, incorporating mindfulness practices can help reduce stress and promote mental health. Engaging with support networks, survivorship groups, and community resources can provide valuable shared experiences, while participating in advocacy efforts can raise awareness and support others facing similar challenges.

Celebrating personal milestones, reflecting on personal growth, and setting realistic goals are important aspects of moving forward in the survivorship journey.

 It is crucial to stay informed about potential long-term effects of treatments and participate in survivorship programs for continued support.

Prioritizing self-care, embracing a holistic approach to wellness, and monitoring and managing any late effects of treatment are essential for maintaining overall health.

Reintegrating into daily life, celebrating personal growth, and connecting with peers for support and mentorship are also important components of the survivorship journey.

Survivorship is a continuous process of adapting, thriving, and maintaining overall well-being after cancer treatment. Embracing the journey with a proactive mindset, accessing available resources, and fostering meaningful connections contribute to a rich and fulfilling life beyond cancer. Each survivor's path is unique, and the collective efforts of individuals, healthcare providers, and support networks contribute to a resilient and empowered survivorship experience.

Chapter 9

Support For Patients And Families

Chaplaincy services offer spiritual care and guidance from chaplains or religious leaders, providing comfort and support to patients and their families.

Additionally, integrating mindfulness and meditation practices as complementary approaches helps support emotional well-being.

Financial assistance programs help individuals navigate the financial burden associated with medical expenses, co-pays, and other related costs. These programs also provide resource referrals for financial counseling and well-being.

Collaboration among healthcare professionals from different disciplines, such as oncologists, nurses, social workers, and other specialists, is crucial in ensuring that patients receive comprehensive and holistic care.

Support groups provide emotional support and a sense of belonging by connecting individuals who are facing similar challenges. Additionally, professional counseling services offer a safe space for individuals and families to address emotional concerns, coping strategies, and communication challenges.

Patient navigation services play a vital role in guiding individuals through the complexities of the healthcare system. These services assist patients in scheduling appointments, understanding treatment plans, and accessing necessary resources.

Recognizing the crucial role of caregivers in the cancer journey, support services such as respite care, counseling, and educational resources are offered to assist and acknowledge their efforts.

Advocacy programs empower patients and families to actively participate in their care and become informed advocates for their needs.

Additionally, involvement in policy advocacy initiatives aims to improve cancer care accessibility, affordability, and overall quality.

Bereavement support services, such as grief counseling and memorial programs, provide assistance and solace to families who have lost a loved one to cancer.

Child life services provide age-appropriate support and activities for pediatric patients, helping them cope with the challenges of cancer treatment. These services also focus on the well-being of the entire family unit, recognizing the impact of cancer on children and parents alike.

Support for patients and families throughout the cancer journey encompasses various aspects, including emotional, psychological, practical, and financial assistance.

Through a network of supportive services, individuals and their families are able to navigate the challenges of cancer with resilience, understanding, and a sense of community.

Workshops on coping strategies, stress management techniques, and resilience-building skills empower patients and families by equipping them with the tools necessary to navigate challenges and uncertainties during the cancer journey.

 Palliative care services focus on relieving symptoms, managing pain, and addressing the emotional and spiritual needs of patients. Early integration of palliative care alongside active treatment ensures overall well-being.

Accessible and reliable educational resources empower patients and families to make informed decisions about their treatment, potential side effects, and survivorship.

Furthermore, workshops and seminars provide opportunities for learning and interacting with healthcare professionals. .

Online communities and telehealth options provide accessible support for patients and families, especially in situations where in-person interaction may be limited. Telehealth platforms also enable remote access to counseling and support services, ensuring continuity of care.

Chapter 10

Advances In Prostate Cancer Research

Targeted therapies have also advanced significantly in prostate cancer research. Androgen receptor signaling inhibitors have been refined, including the development of second-generation inhibitors, expanding treatment options for patients.

Additionally, the emerging role of poly(ADP-ribose) polymerase (PARP) inhibitors in treating prostate cancers with DNA repair deficiencies has shown great potential in improving patient outcomes.

Liquid biopsy and circulating tumor DNA analysis have emerged as non-invasive monitoring techniques in prostate cancer research.

Liquid biopsy techniques allow for the detection of circulating tumor DNA, facilitating non-invasive monitoring of disease progression and treatment response.

This breakthrough offers the potential for earlier detection of recurrence or metastasis, leading to timely interventions and better patient outcomes.

Immunotherapy has emerged as a promising avenue in prostate cancer research. Immune checkpoint inhibitors, such as PD-1/PD-L1 inhibitors, have shown great potential in activating the immune system against prostate cancer cells. This breakthrough has opened up new possibilities for treating advanced prostate cancer and improving patient outcomes.

Furthermore, the investigational use of chimeric antigen receptor (CAR) T-cell therapy for targeting prostate cancer cells has shown promise and is currently being studied extensively.

Advancements in imaging technologies have revolutionized the way prostate cancer is visualized and diagnosed. PSMA-PET imaging, utilizing prostate-specific membrane antigen PET scans, offers improved precision in detecting and staging prostate cancer. This technology has significantly enhanced the accuracy of diagnosis and treatment planning.

Similarly, enhancements in MRI technology, specifically multiparametric MRI (mpMRI), have contributed to more accurate visualization of prostate tumors, leading to better treatment decisions and improved patient outcomes.

Theranostics and radioisotope therapy have shown great promise in prostate cancer research. PSMA theranostics, which integrate diagnostic imaging with therapeutic interventions targeting PSMA-positive prostate cancer cells, have shown great potential in improving treatment outcomes.

Additionally, the investigational use of Lutetium-177 PSMA therapy, a radioisotope therapy for advanced prostate cancer treatment, is currently being studied extensively, and early results are promising.

In conclusion, advances in prostate cancer research have led to significant advancements in Precision Medicine and Biomarkers, Immunotherapy, Targeted Therapies, Imaging Technologies, Liquid Biopsy and Circulating Tumor DNA, Theranostics and Radioisotope Therapy, and Microbiome Research.

These breakthroughs offer hope to patients and healthcare professionals, revolutionizing the way prostate cancer is diagnosed, treated, and monitored.

Further research and clinical trials are needed to fully harness the potential of these advancements and improve patient outcomes in the fight against prostate cancer.

Precision Medicine and Biomarkers have played a crucial role in prostate cancer research.

Genomic profiling has allowed researchers to identify specific genetic mutations and alterations in prostate cancer cells, leading to a better understanding of the disease.

Additionally, the development of more accurate biomarkers has improved early detection, risk stratification, and personalized treatment planning, allowing for more targeted and effective therapies.

Advances in Prostate Cancer Research have led to significant breakthroughs in various areas, including Precision Medicine and Biomarkers, Immunotherapy, Targeted Therapies, Imaging Technologies, Liquid Biopsy and Circulating Tumor DNA, Theranostics and Radioisotope Therapy, and Microbiome Research. These advancements have revolutionized the way prostate cancer is diagnosed, treated, and monitored, offering hope to patients and healthcare professionals.

 Microbiome research has also gained attention in prostate cancer research. The study of the microbiome, the collection of microorganisms residing in the body, has revealed potential links between the microbiome and prostate cancer development and progression. Understanding the role of the microbiome in prostate cancer may lead to innovative treatment approaches and personalized interventions.

Overall, the advancements in prostate cancer research are transforming our understanding of the disease and driving the development of innovative therapeutic approaches. From precision medicine to immunotherapy breakthroughs and the integration of artificial intelligence, ongoing research endeavors hold immense potential to revolutionize prostate cancer care, ultimately leading to improved outcomes for individuals affected by this complex disease.

Epigenetic modifications play a significant role in prostate cancer development, and research in this area provides insights into how these alterations contribute to the disease. Investigating targeted therapies aimed at modifying epigenetic processes holds promise for therapeutic benefit.

The integration of artificial intelligence (AI) is revolutionizing prostate cancer research. The use of AI in radiomics enhances the analysis of imaging data, leading to more precise diagnosis and treatment planning.

AI-assisted tools contribute to treatment decision support by analyzing complex datasets and identifying patterns.

Understanding tumor heterogeneity is another crucial aspect of prostate cancer research.

Advancements in single-cell sequencing technologies allow for a comprehensive understanding of the diversity within tumors. Exploring intra-tumoral variability helps in developing targeted therapeutic strategies to address the different populations of cancer cells.

Collaborative research initiatives are vital in accelerating the pace of discovery and innovation in prostate cancer research. Global collaborations between research institutions, pharmaceutical companies, and advocacy groups facilitate the sharing of data and promote a more comprehensive understanding of prostate cancer biology.

The exploration of the gut microbiome's influence on prostate cancer development, progression, and treatment response is an area of great interest in current research.

There is a focus on investigating strategies to modulate the microbiome for potential therapeutic benefits. Ongoing clinical trials are exploring innovative treatment modalities, including novel drug combinations and therapeutic approaches.

Patient-centric research is also gaining importance, incorporating individual patient characteristics to develop personalized treatment strategies.

Artificial intelligence (AI) is revolutionizing the field of pathology and its application in prostate cancer research holds great promise. AI algorithms can analyze large volumes of pathology data with great accuracy and efficiency, aiding in the diagnosis and classification of prostate cancer.

This technology has the potential to improve decision-making, optimize treatment strategies, and contribute to personalized medicine in the field of prostate cancer.

Researchers are also exploring the influence of metabolic alterations in prostate cancer and potential therapeutic interventions targeting metabolic pathways.

This area of study, known as metabolic reprogramming, aims to understand how changes in metabolic processes contribute to the development and progression of prostate cancer.

Additionally, the impact of dietary interventions such as ketogenic diets and intermittent fasting on prostate cancer metabolism is being investigated.

One area of promising research in the field of prostate cancer is the development of investigational androgen receptor degraders (ARDs) utilizing proteolysis-targeting chimeras (PROTAC) technology. These ARDs, such as ARV-110, show potential in overcoming resistance to traditional hormonal therapies.

Additionally, selective androgen receptor degraders (SARDs) are being developed with the goal of more targeted and effective disruption of androgen receptor signaling.

With the ongoing global health landscape and the need for enhanced patient care, the implementation of telehealth and remote monitoring technologies has become increasingly important. Remote patient monitoring allows healthcare providers to monitor patients' health status from a distance, enabling timely interventions and reducing the need for in-person visits.

Similarly, virtual clinical trials are being explored as a way to increase accessibility and participant engagement by leveraging digital platforms.

In order to assess the impact of treatment on quality of life, there is a growing emphasis on incorporating patient-reported outcomes into prostate cancer research. This comprehensive assessment takes into account the patients' perspectives and experiences, providing valuable insights into the effectiveness of different treatments and interventions.

Furthermore, there is a movement towards integrating holistic care measures into research, addressing not only the physical aspects of well-being but also the psychological and social aspects.

AI pathology is the integration of artificial intelligence technology into the field of pathology, which is the study of diseases and their effects on the human body. This innovative approach utilizes machine learning algorithms and computer vision techniques to analyze medical images, such as tissue samples and scans, in order to assist pathologists in diagnosing and interpreting diseases more accurately and efficiently.

By harnessing the power of AI, pathology is being revolutionized, leading to improved diagnostic accuracy, faster turnaround times, and ultimately better patient outcomes. This cutting-edge technology has the potential to transform the way diseases are detected and treated, making it an exciting development in the field of medicine.

Conclusion

In conclusion, the landscape of prostate cancer is continually evolving, shaped by advances in research, treatment modalities, and a growing understanding of risk factors. This comprehensive exploration of prostate cancer, spanning from understanding the disease and its nuances to prevention strategies and the latest in research, underscores the importance of a holistic approach to prostate health.

As we navigate the complexities of prostate cancer, it becomes evident that individualized care, early detection, and proactive prevention are crucial elements in improving outcomes. From lifestyle modifications to innovative therapies, this journey involves collaboration between individuals, healthcare providers, researchers, supportive communities.

While significant progress has been made in prostate cancer research and care, challenges persist. Addressing disparities in access to care, refining screening approaches, and further unraveling the complexities of tumor heterogeneity are ongoing priorities. The integration of patient-centric care, personalized treatment plans, and the incorporation of cutting-edge technologies contribute to a more hopeful and informed approach to managing prostate cancer.

In the realm of prevention, empowering individuals with knowledge about lifestyle choices, genetic factors, and early detection measures is pivotal. Proactive efforts, such as maintaining a healthy lifestyle, routine screenings, and risk assessments, can play a crucial role in reducing the burden of prostate cancer.

As we look toward the future, continued collaboration, advocacy, and research endeavors will be instrumental in furthering our understanding of prostate cancer and refining treatment approaches. Empowering individuals with information, fostering a supportive environment, and advancing scientific discoveries collectively contribute to the overarching goal of improving the lives of those affected by prostate cancer.

In this dynamic landscape, the collective efforts of healthcare professionals, researchers, patients, and their families shape the trajectory of prostate cancer care. By embracing a comprehensive and multidisciplinary approach, we move closer to a future where prostate cancer is not just treated but prevented, managed, and ultimately conquered.

As we move forward, it is imperative to emphasize the role of education and awareness in promoting early detection and proactive health management. Encouraging regular check-ups, advocating for healthy lifestyles, and fostering open dialogues about prostate health contribute to a culture of preventive care.

The dynamic interplay of science, technology, and compassionate patient care defines the ongoing narrative of prostate cancer. Research breakthroughs, such as precision medicine, immunotherapy, and advanced imaging technologies, hold the promise of more targeted and effective treatments. Moreover, the exploration of preventive measures, genetic insights, and lifestyle interventions positions us on the brink of transformative strides in prostate cancer prevention.

In conclusion, the journey through prostate cancer encompasses a spectrum of experiences, from understanding the intricacies of the disease to navigating treatment options and embracing preventive measures. The resilience of individuals facing prostate cancer, coupled with the dedication of healthcare professionals and the advancements in research, paints a hopeful picture for the future.

As we stand at the intersection of knowledge and innovation, let us continue to champion progress in prostate cancer care. By fostering a collaborative and supportive ecosystem, we lay the foundation for a future where prostate cancer is not only treatable but preventable, and where each individual's journey is characterized by empowerment, dignity, and optimal quality of life. Together, we can shape a future where prostate health is prioritized, and the impact of this complex disease is minimized for generations to come.

Acknowledgement

I wish to thank Almighty God for the inspiration to undertake this project and contribute to the society positively.

About the Author

Leo Chambers is a creative writer and Digital Content Creator.

9 798883 714640